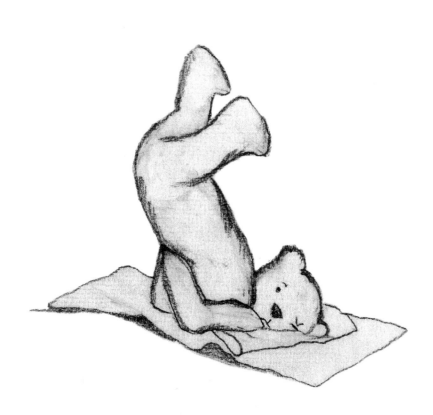

Yoga for Bears

YOGA
for
BEARS

A Little Primer on the Unbearable Rightness of Bending

Rosamond Richardson *and* James Ward

HarperSanFrancisco
A Division of HarperCollins*Publishers*

*For Lucy and William
with thanks to Chantek, Françoise, and Robin*

YOGA FOR BEARS: *A Little Primer on the Unbearable Rightness of Bending.*
Copyright © 1995 by Rosamond Richardson and James Ward. All rights
reserved. Printed in the United States of America. No part of this book
may be used or reproduced in any manner whatsoever without written
permission except in the case of brief quotations embodied in critical
articles and reviews. For information address HarperCollins *Publishers,* 10
East 53rd Street, New York, NY 10022.

FIRST EDITION

Library of Congress Cataloging-in-Publication Data

Richardson, Rosamond. 1945–
  [Yoga for beginner bears]
  Yoga for bears : a little primer on the unbearable rightness of bending /
  Rosamond Richardson and James Ward. — 1st ed.
    p. cm.
  Originally published in Great Britain by Ebury Press under the title :
  Yoga for beginner bears.
  ISBN 0–06–251182–3
  ISBN 0–06–251181–5 (pbk.)
  1. Yoga, Hatha I. Ward, James. II. Title
RA781.7.R54   1995
613.8'046—dc20   94–34777
                                          CIP

---

95 96 97 98 99 HAD 10 9 8 7 6 5 4 3 2 1

This edition is printed on acid-free paper that meets the American
National Standards Institute Z39.48 Standard.

Contents

Yoga For Bears

What is Yoga?

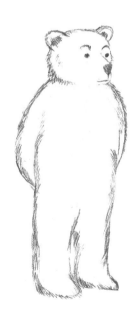

'Yoga', said the second-century sage Patanjali, 'is the stilling of the thought-waves of the mind.' Inner serenity, evenness and clarity are cultivated through the training and practice of various disciplines. One of these is 'hatha yoga', a form of exercise that puts the body in touch with its connection to other levels of being – mental, emotional and spiritual.

In ancient India wise men devised countless bodily postures to refine and energize the body. These postures, known as hatha yoga, are still practised all over the world today. They all have Sanskrit names, some of which relate to nature – animals, birds, plants or landscape, some to familiar objects, and others to heroes and gods. These names all end in 'asana' – the Sanskrit name for posture or position.

The word 'yoga' means 'union' – a union of the human soul with the spiritual ground of its being, that 'universal spirit' which is known by different names in different cultures. The Bhagavad Gita, an immortal Sanskrit poem of light, love and life, written in the fifth century BC and still an inspiration to yogis today, describes each individual soul as being a spark of that immense universal spirit.

'Practise becomes firmly grounded', says Patanjali, 'when it has been cultivated for a long time, uninterruptedly, with earnest devotion.' And the result of this practice? The words of the Bhagavad

Gita tell us that 'In this union of yoga there is liberty: a deliverance from the oppression of pain. This Yoga must be followed with faith, with a strong courageous heart'.

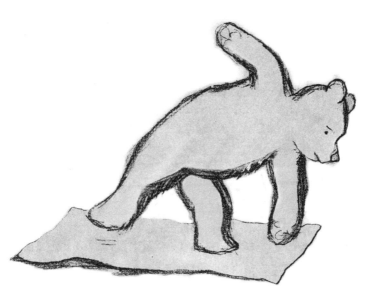

Why Practise Yoga?

The practice of yoga postures has the effect of not only calming the mind and centering the soul, it makes the body feel really good too. You become stronger, more supple, more co-ordinated. You feel healthy, young and radiant. You become more aware of your body and how it works, and you educate it in new ways. You are more in touch with gravity and with how you breathe. The postures energize and refresh rather than tire you. The body responds with joy to the positions; so to practise yoga is to enjoy yourself, stretch your body pleasurably, calm your mind and resume your everyday life with a sense of well-being.

'Yoga is a harmony. Not for him who eats too much, or for him who eats too little; not for him who sleeps too little, or for him who sleeps too much.'

'A harmony is eating and resting, in sleeping and keeping awake: a perfection in whatever one does. This is the Yoga that gives peace from all pain.'
Bhagavad Gita

YOGA IS EVENNESS OF MIND – A PEACE THAT IS EVER THE SAME.

Hints and Advice

Always leave two hours after eating a full meal
before you practise.

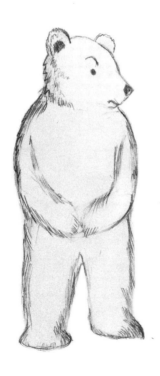

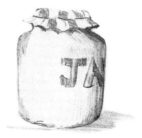

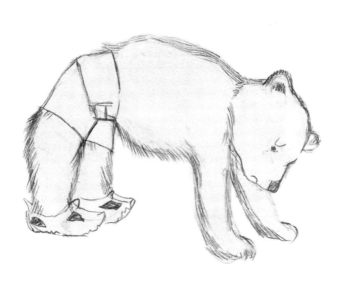

Wear loose clothing and work in bare feet.

Use a non-slip mat to prevent accidental strain or injury. Some poses, like headstands, are helped by a folded blanket.

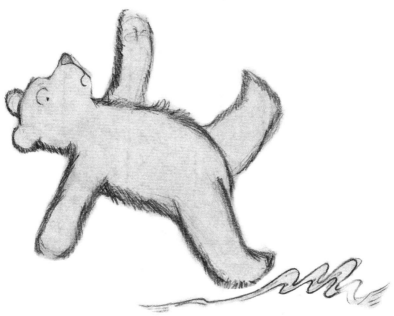

Go carefully! Some of the poses are very strong. Hold the poses for a short time only, for as long as you can hold them without strain until your body gets used to them.

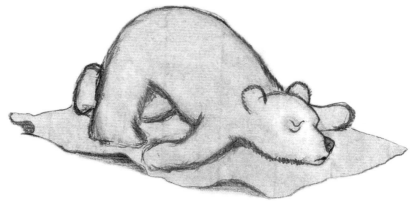

If you want to learn the postures properly, find a good teacher and go to a regular class.

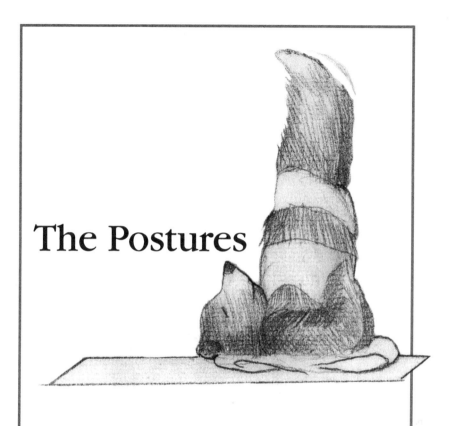

The Postures

'Do thy work in the peace of Yoga and, free from
selfish desires, be not moved by success or failure.
Yoga is evenness of mind.'
Bhagavad Gita

Legs up the Wall
Viparita korani
This position aligns the entire body and gives a
wonderful rest to the back.

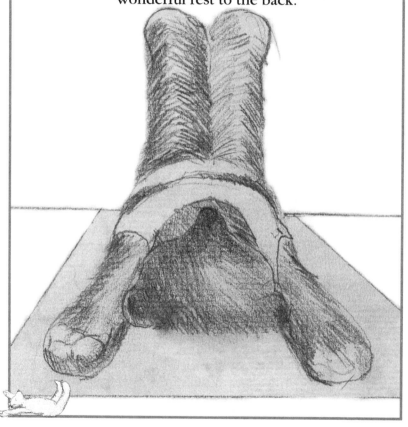

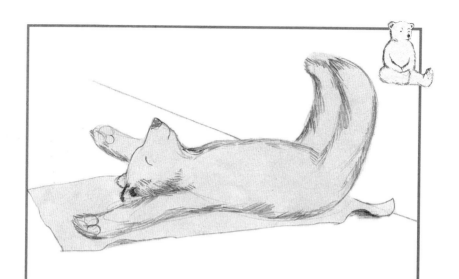

All the muscles in the trunk, from the neck down to the pelvis, relax deeply. The legs are well rested. Five to ten minutes in this position completely restores flagging energy. It is a useful pose at the beginning of a practice session as it softens the body and quietens the mind.

Salute to the Sun
Urdhva hastasana
This is the first movement of the well-known 'Salute to the Sun'.

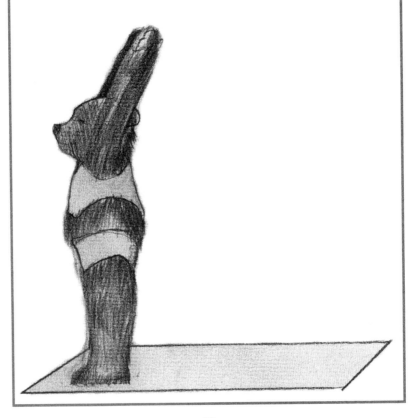

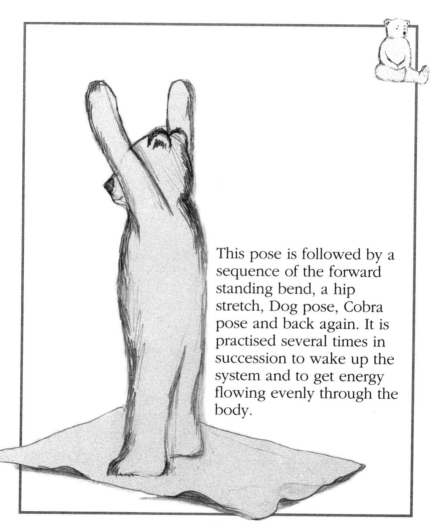

This pose is followed by a sequence of the forward standing bend, a hip stretch, Dog pose, Cobra pose and back again. It is practised several times in succession to wake up the system and to get energy flowing evenly through the body.

Dog Pose
Adho mukha svanasana
This exhilarating pose relieves fatigue, rejuvenates the brain cells and renews energy.

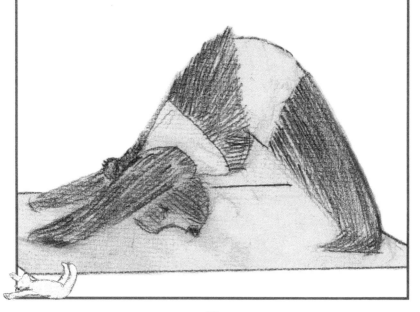

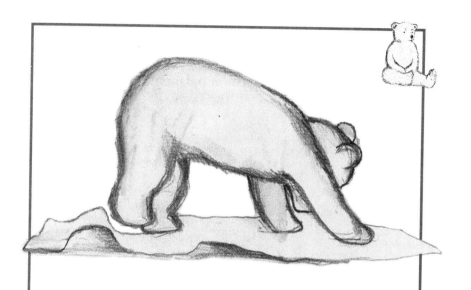

The pose resembles a dog stretching its forelegs with its head down and hindquarters up. The hands are pressed firmly into the floor with the fingers spread evenly, the arms are fully stretched and the trunk extended. The hamstrings are stretched as the backs of the knees open.

Tree

Vrksasana

This pose brings a sense of balance, stillness and poise to the body.

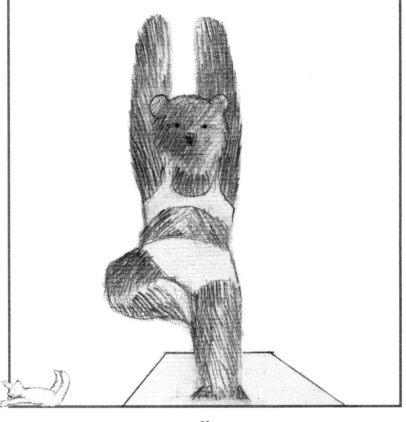

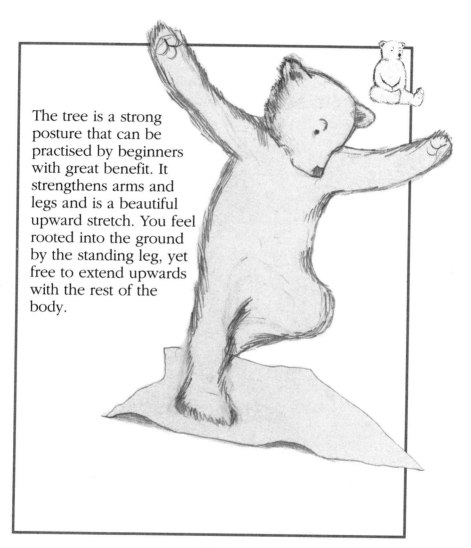

The tree is a strong posture that can be practised by beginners with great benefit. It strengthens arms and legs and is a beautiful upward stretch. You feel rooted into the ground by the standing leg, yet free to extend upwards with the rest of the body.

Standing Forward-Stretch
Uttanasana
There is a wonderful feeling of calm after doing this pose.

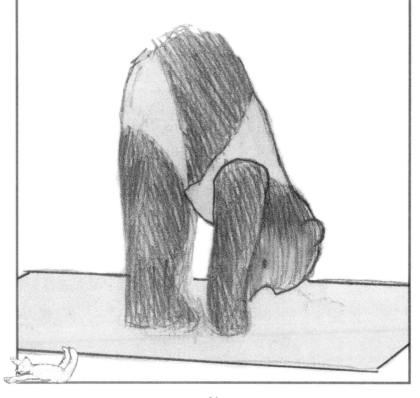

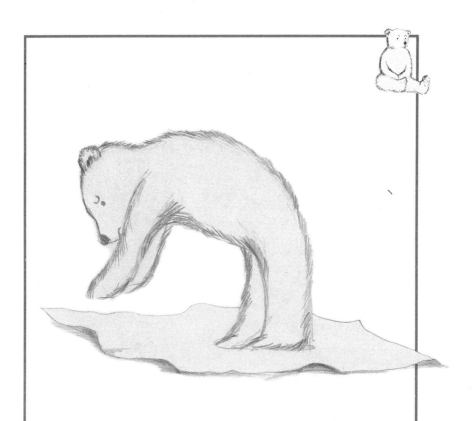

This intense extension of the spine forwards over the
legs gives the back a deliberate stretch and loosens
the hips. It tones internal organs, slows the heartbeat,
rejuvenates spinal nerves, and soothes the brain cells.

Triangle
Trikonasana

Both stability and a good sense of balance are increased by this pose.

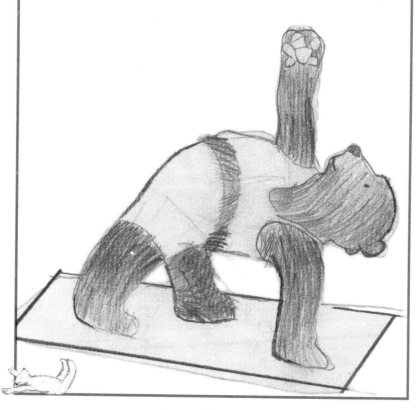

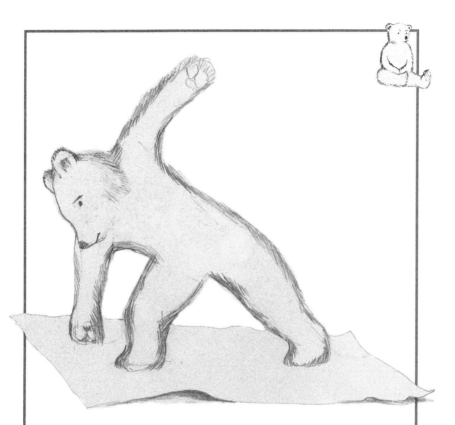

The triangle posture tones the leg muscles and relieves stiffness in both legs and hips. It is good for backache and a strained neck, and opens up the chest. The well-grounded feet connect the body with gravity.

Powerful Pose
Utkatasana
This position is like sitting down on
an imaginary chair.

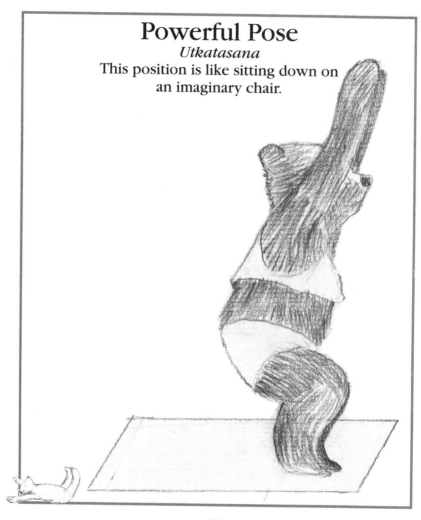

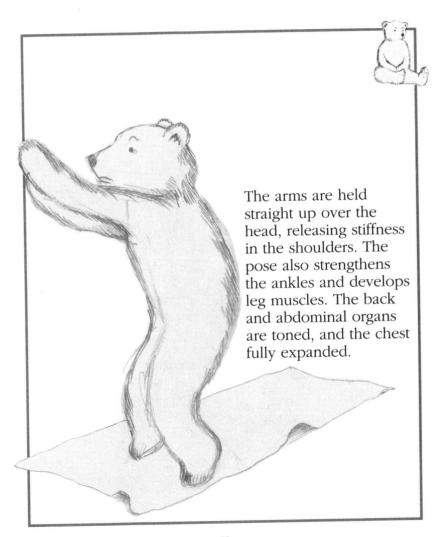

The arms are held straight up over the head, releasing stiffness in the shoulders. The pose also strengthens the ankles and develops leg muscles. The back and abdominal organs are toned, and the chest fully expanded.

Head to Knee (Standing)
Padangusthasana
The abdominal organs are toned and gastric troubles relieved by this pose.

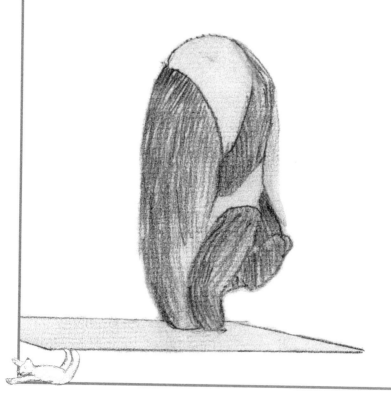

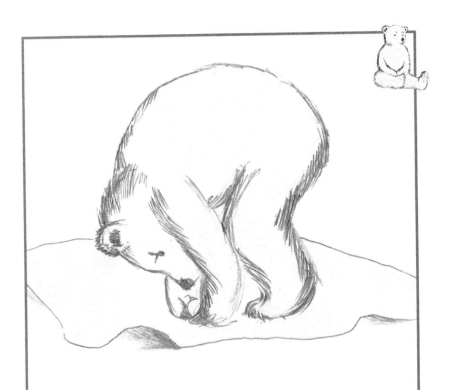

This posture is performed standing, bending down to catch the big toes without bending the knees. Look up at first, then stretch down to bring the head towards the knees. It extends the hamstrings and stretches the spine, as well as loosening the hips.

Warrior Pose II
Virabhadrasana II
For all its apparent simplicity, this is a challenging
pose to practise correctly.

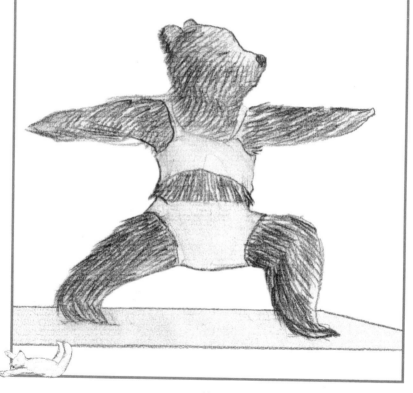

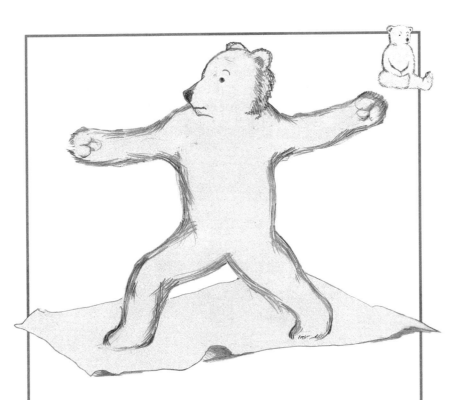

Human geometry in action, this pose aligns the trunk to the vertical, the arms and front thigh to the horizontal. The posture shapes and tones leg muscles, releases the muscles in the back, and tones the abdominal organs.

Warrior Pose III
Virabhadrasana III
This last of three Warrior poses shows the harmony,
balance and poise that can be attained in yoga.

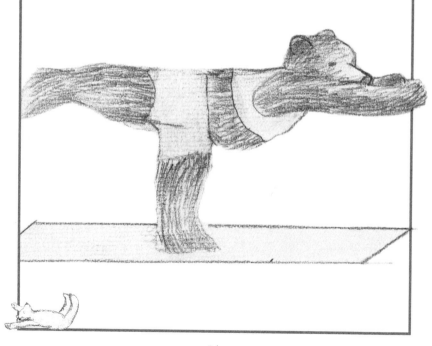

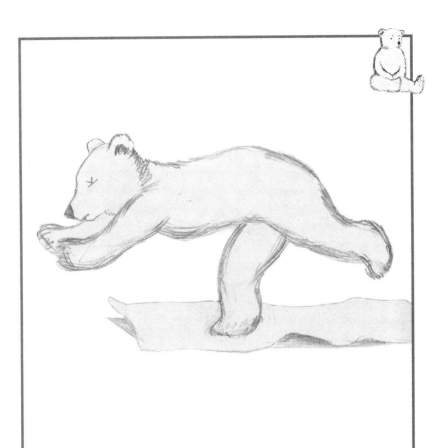

This position is recommended for runners as it develops vigour and co-ordination, and strengthens leg muscles. It helps one to stand firmly on the soles of the feet, and brings agility to body and mind.

Half Moon
Ardha chandrasana
A sense of freedom is experienced when you practise this pose well.

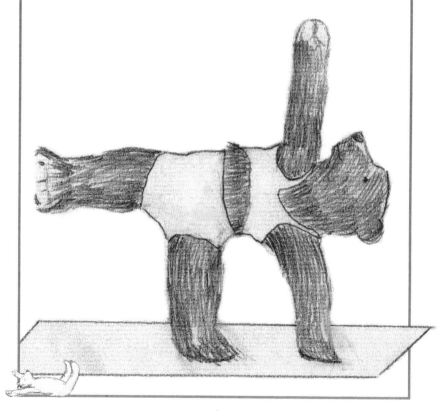

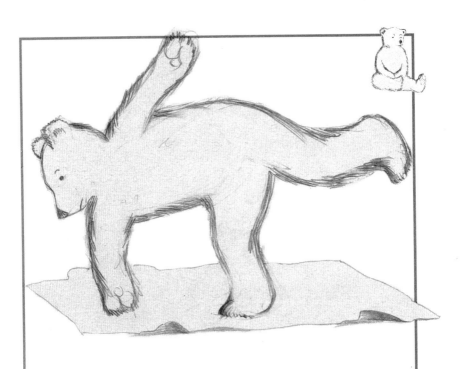

This balance teaches the body poise and stability. It tones the lower spine and strengthens the legs, particularly the knees. By practising the co-ordination involved in this posture, the body will develop grace and rhythm.

Bridge
Setu bandha
This pose is useful for beginners, introducing the
body to back-bending gently and pleasantly.

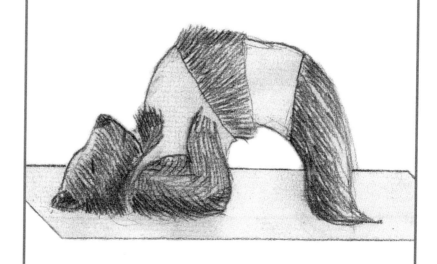

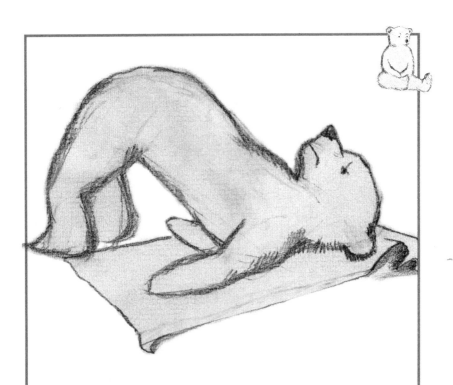

Here the body is arched over from shoulder to heels, supported by the hands under the waist. The posture makes the spine healthy and flexible, toning the nervous system. It is a pleasant stretch for the neck and shoulders. After mastering this pose, move on to more difficult postures like The Wheel.

The East
Purvottasana
The entire front of the body (the 'east') is stretched
from the forehead to the toes.

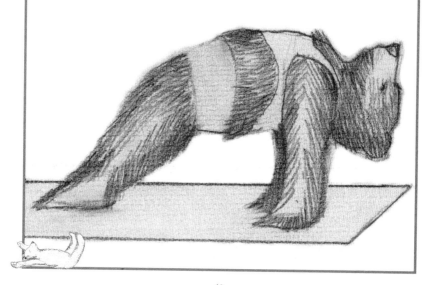

This pose strengthens the wrists and ankles, improves mobility in the shoulder joints, and expands the chest fully. The legs get a good stretch and the feet are brought to life by being extended until the toes touch the floor.

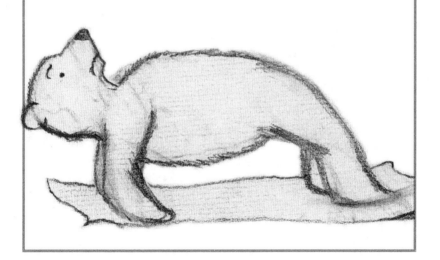

Cobra Pose
Bhujangasana
This position tones the entire spine and relieves a stiff back.

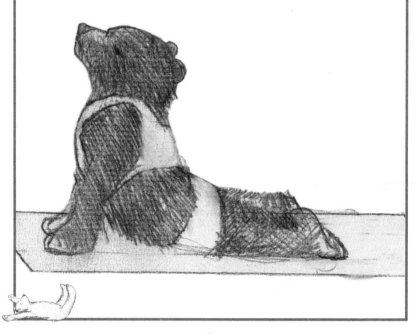

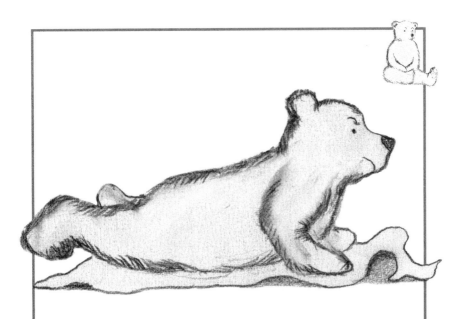

In this pose the body resembles a serpent about to strike. The head is thrown back, the chest expanded and the legs fully stretched. This back bend is to be done gently and carefully, using the breathing to facilitate the stretch. Stay in it for a short period only, and lie on your front afterwards before repeating it.

Camel
Ustrasana
The Camel can be practised by beginners and the elderly.

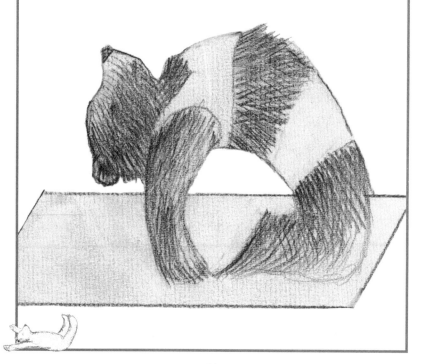

Kneeling and leaning back to hold the heels, with the hips pushed forward, the whole spine is stretched backwards and toned. The posture opens up the shoulders, and corrects a rounded back. It is important to keep the eyes soft and the neck relaxed as you look back, and to come up evenly and slowly.

Headstand
Sirsasana
The headstand is the King to the shoulderstand's
Queen.

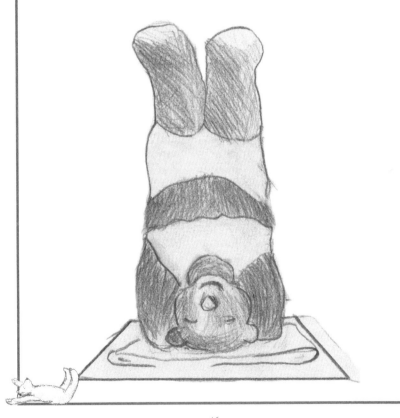

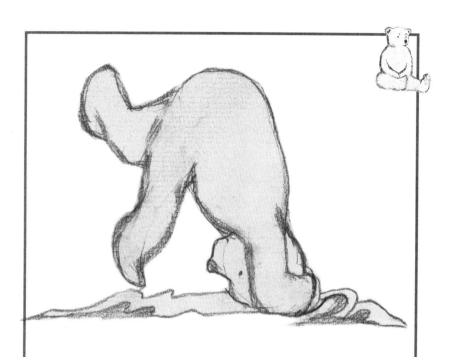

Along with the shoulderstand, the headstand is one of the most important postures in yoga. Mastery of the headstand gives both physical and mental balance and poise. The practice keeps the body healthy and the mind tranquil and peaceful. It is not a posture for beginners to do on their own, since it requires strength, guidance and practice.

Shoulderstand
Sarvangasana
The whole body benefits from this pose, which is
often practised after the headstand.

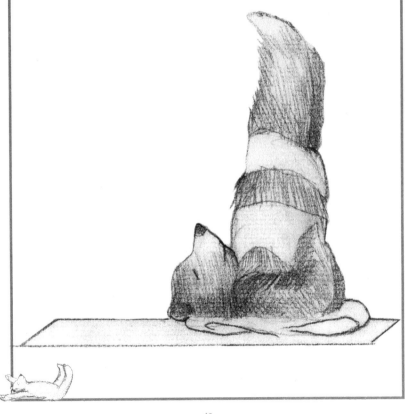

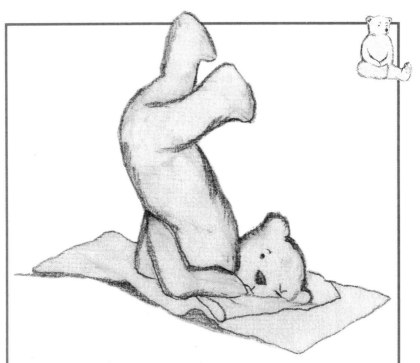

The shoulderstand brings harmony to the system and is a panacea for common ailments, hence it has been called the Queen of the Asanas. The shoulderstand regulates glandular secretion and soothes the nerves. The change in bodily gravity eliminates toxins from the system and increases vitality by refreshing major internal organs. It brings new vigour and strength, resulting in a feeling of well-being and confidence.

Shoulderstand Variation
Eka pada sarvangasana
This posture tones the kidneys and the leg muscles.

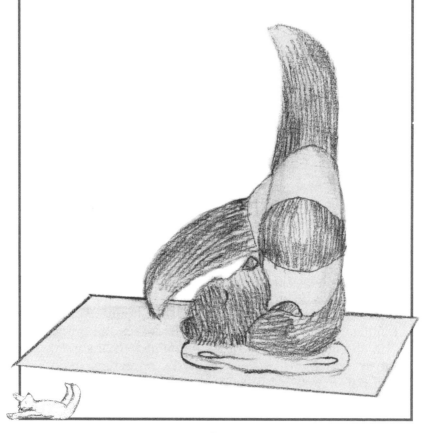

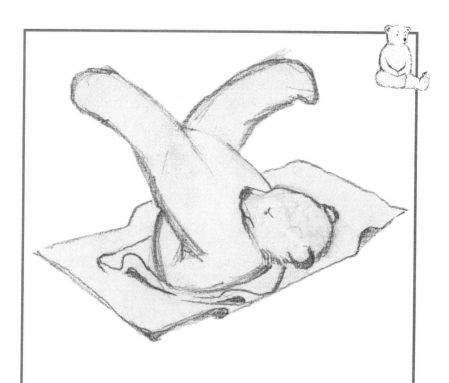

In this variation, one leg comes down to the floor as in the Plough, while the other is kept in a line vertical with the trunk. This pose also brings the benefits of all inverted postures: refreshing the brain and internal organs, revitalizing the circulation, and resting the legs.

Plough
Halasana
This is a restful pose and can be done with the legs
supported on a chair.

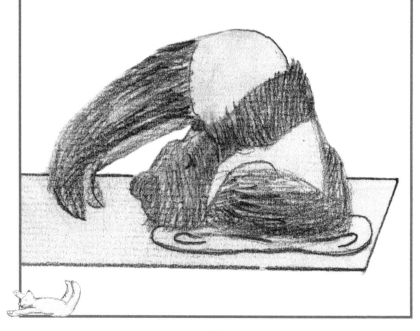

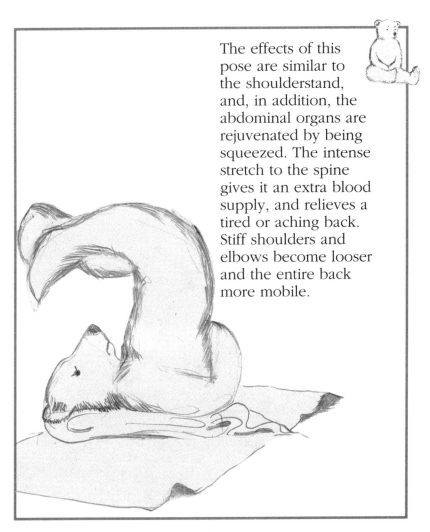

The effects of this pose are similar to the shoulderstand, and, in addition, the abdominal organs are rejuvenated by being squeezed. The intense stretch to the spine gives it an extra blood supply, and relieves a tired or aching back. Stiff shoulders and elbows become looser and the entire back more mobile.

Plough Variation
Supta konasana
This variation rests the heart and soothes the
nervous system.

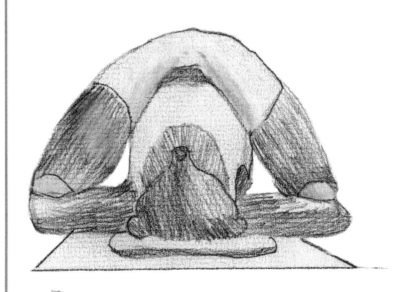

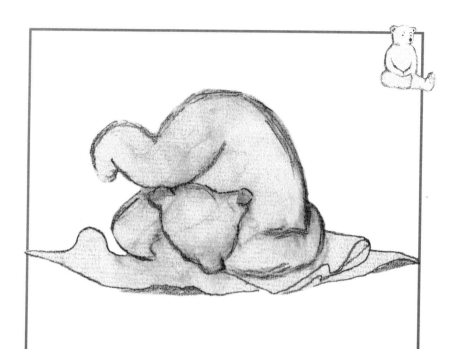

In addition to the benefits of the plough pose, this variation tones the legs and helps contract the abdominal organs. From the plough position, the legs are taken wide apart and the hands hold the feet.

The Wheel
Urdhva dhanurasana
This is not a posture for beginners as it requires
considerable strength and flexibility.

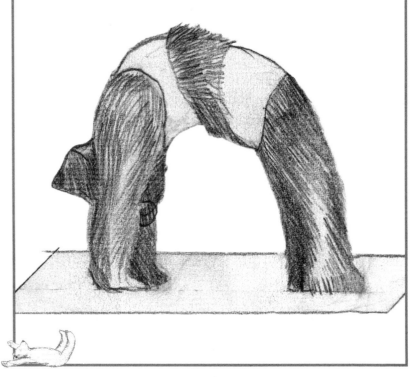

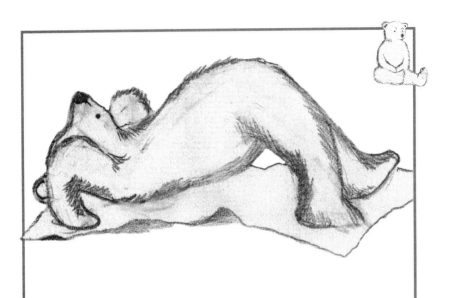

In this back arch the spine is fully toned and the body brought to a state of alert suppleness. You feel strong and full of life after practising it. Arms and wrists are strengthened, and it gives you increased vitality, energy and a feeling of lightness.

Handstand
Adho mukha vrksasana
A strong gymnastic pose, this arm-balance develops the body harmoniously.

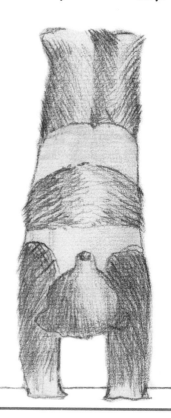

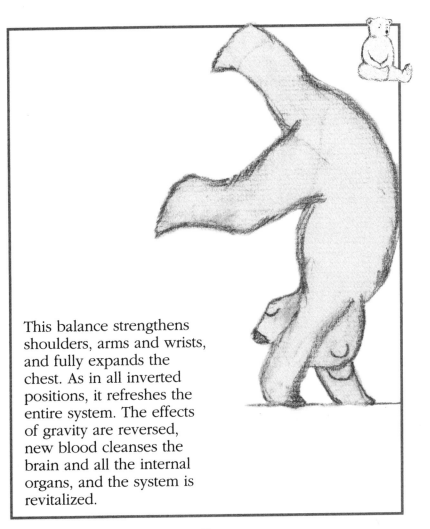

This balance strengthens
shoulders, arms and wrists,
and fully expands the
chest. As in all inverted
positions, it refreshes the
entire system. The effects
of gravity are reversed,
new blood cleanses the
brain and all the internal
organs, and the system is
revitalized.

The Rod
Dandasana
Dandasana is the starting point for all the seated
forward-bending postures.

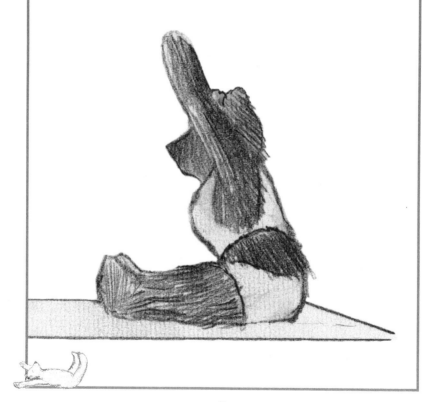

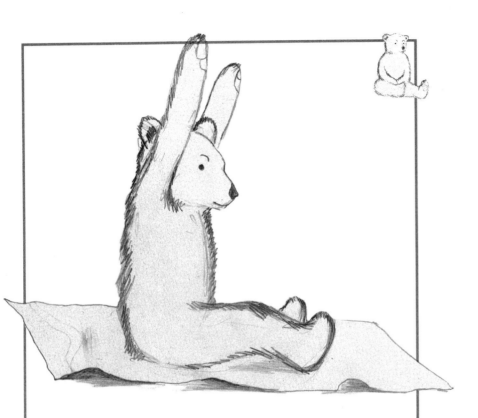

The rod or staff posture aligns the spine correctly for an upright sitting position, and stretches the legs fully. The hips are lifted so that you are sitting on your sitting-bones, the spine is released upwards and the top chest opens.

Boat
Navasana
This pose enables the body to grow old gracefully
and comfortably.

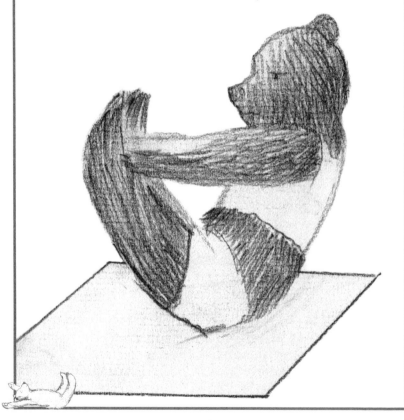

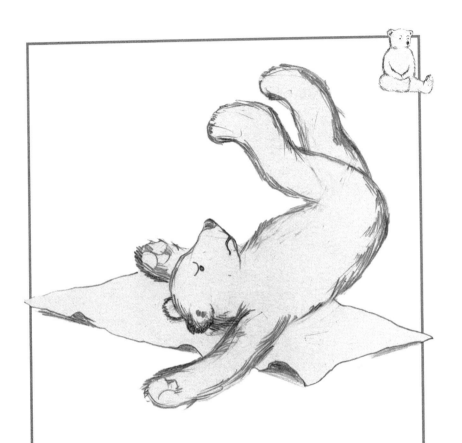

So-called because the pose looks like the shape of a boat, this posture acts strongly on the intestines, liver and spleen. It helps to strengthen the spine and brings life and vigour to the back.

Head to Knee (Sitting)
Janu sirsasana
This is a good pose to do if you are running
a low fever.

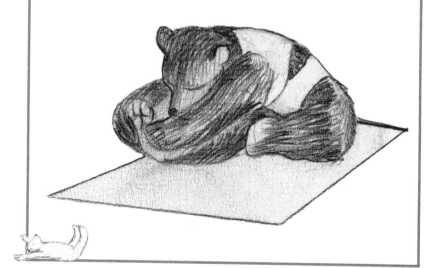

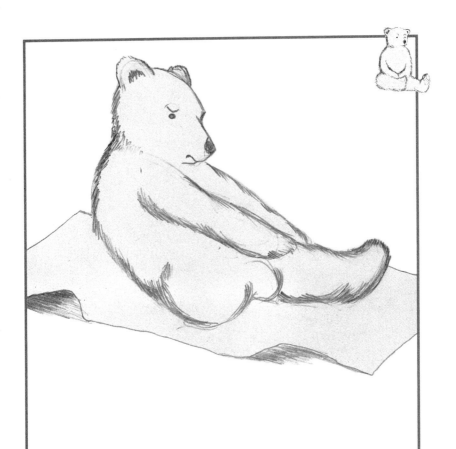

In this posture one leg is stretched out in front, the other is bent at the knee and taken in to the side. Bending forward to put head to knee tones the liver and spleen and also activates the kidneys.

Forward Bend

Paschimottanasana

'Paschima' means the 'west' and this position
stretches the back of the body.

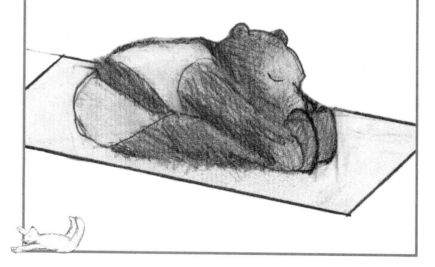

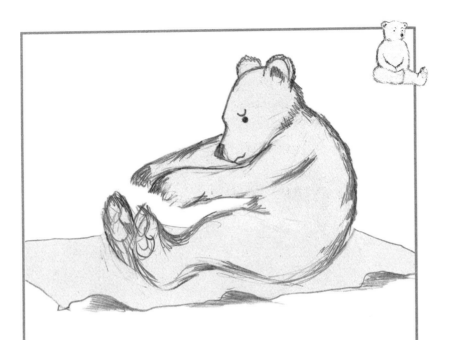

The 'west' side of the body, the back, is powerfully
stretched from the head to the heels. The whole
spine is rejuvenated by this pose, which also tones
the kidneys and improves the digestion. The nervous
system is toned and soothed, the mind rested and
overall vitality increased as a result of practising
this pose.

Sitting Twist
Marichyasana III
Marichyasana III is one of yoga's most classical and
statuesque of poses.

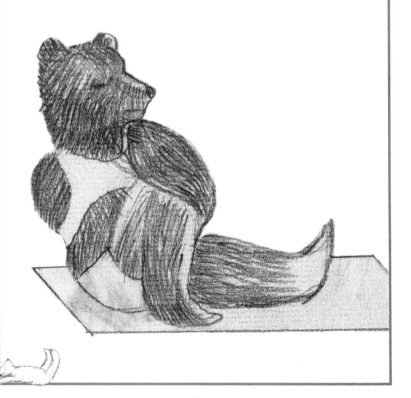

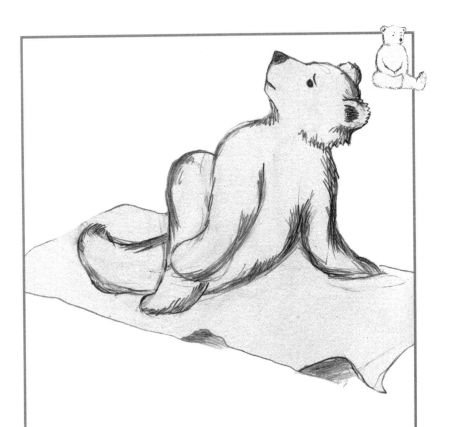

Sitting twists have a cleansing effect on the system. Backache, lumbago and pain in the hips disappear rapidly by the regular practice of this twist. The liver, spleen and intestines also benefit, while shoulder movements become freer and the neck stronger.

Sitting Twist II
Ardha matsyendrasana
The shoulders are loosened by the practice of this posture, and the upper back released.

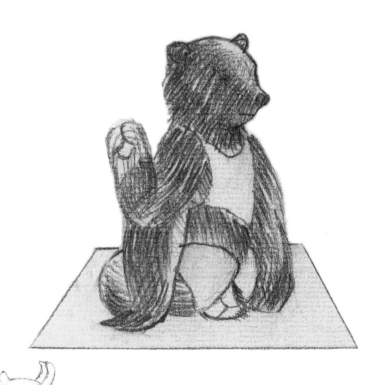

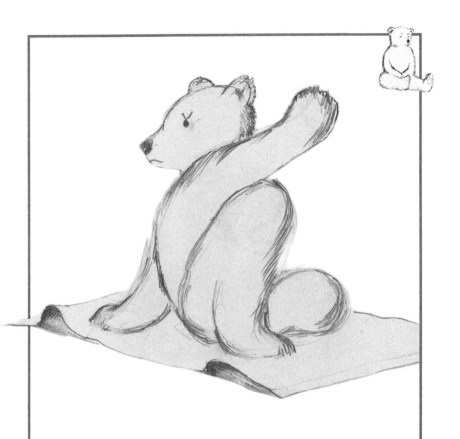

Matsyendra was the Lord of the Fishes, who
overheard Lord Siva explaining the mysteries of yoga
to his consort Parvati. Here the spine is given a mild
lateral twist, and the abdomen is squeezed.

Cobbler Pose
Baddha konasana
Indian cobblers traditionally sit in this position.

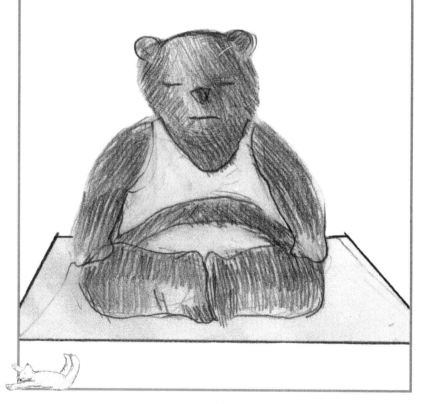

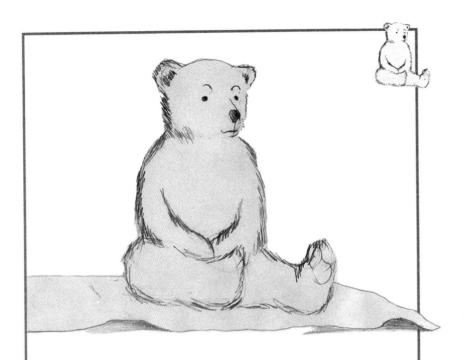

The pose stimulates the pelvic region and the abdomen, and keeps the bladder and kidneys healthy. It is a blessing to women as it stretches the pelvic floor, helps the ovaries to function properly and checks irregular menstrual cycles. This pose is sometimes used for meditation, and can be practised after a meal without discomfort.

Lotus Pose
Padmasana
The Buddha is often depicted sitting in the lotus pose.

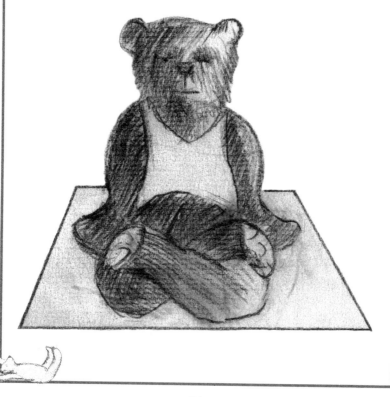

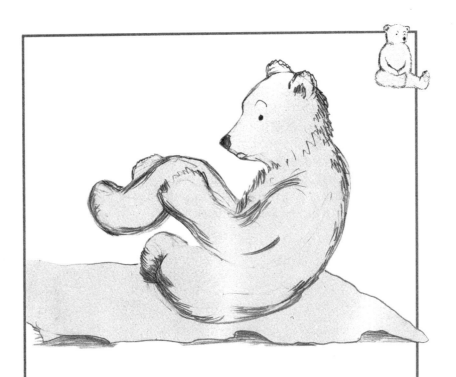

The lotus is one of the most important and useful postures in yoga, and when mastered is ideal for meditation. It is an advanced pose as it requires considerable mobility in the hips, knees and feet.

Corpse Pose
Savasana

A yoga practice is completed by lying on the floor, the body aligned, legs rolling apart and arms slightly away from the body with the palms of the hands facing up. The head can be supported by a low pillow. Relaxing deeply with the eyes closed, centering with the breathing, this pose integrates the work of the postures and brings the body and mind to a state of deep peace and stillness.

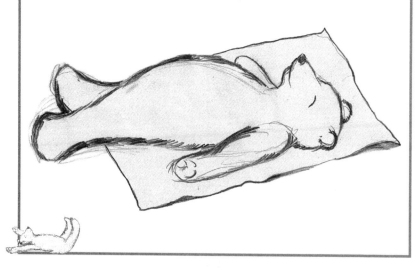

'And a man should not abandon his work, even if he cannot achieve it in full perfection; because in all work there may be imperfection, even as in all fire there is smoke.'

'When in the Yoga of holy contemplation the movements of the mind and of the breath of life are in a harmony of peace, there is steadiness, and that steadiness is pure.'
Bhagavad Gita

Recommended Reading

Iyengar, B. K. S. *Light on Yoga*. New York: Schocken, 1987.

Iyengar, B. K. S. *Light on the Yoga Sutras of Patanjali*. San Francisco: Aquarian, 1993.

Mascaro, Juan, trans. *Bhagavad Gita*. New York: Viking Penguin, 1962.

Mascaro, Juan, trans. *Dhammapada*. New York: Viking Penguin, 1973.

Mascaro, Juan, trans. *Upanishads*. New York: Viking Penguin, 1965.

Mehta, Mira and Shyam. *Yoga the Iyengar Way*. New York: Knopf, 1990.

O'Brien, Paddy. *Yoga for Women*. San Francisco: Aquarian, 1994.

Scaravelli, Vanda. *Awakening the Spine*. San Francisco: Harper San Francisco, 1991.

Stewart, Mary and Kathy Phillips. *Yoga for Children*. New York: Simon & Schuster Trade, 1993.

Weller, Stella and W. Harry Gahrni. *The Yoga Back Book*. San Francisco: Thorsons San Francisco, 1993.

Useful addresses for finding a Yoga class

B. K. S. Iyengar Yoga National Association
8223 West 3rd Street
Los Angeles, CA 90038

Iyengar Yoga Institute of San Francisco
2404 27th Avenue at Taraval Street
San Francisco, CA 94116

Kripalu Center for Yoga and Health
Box 793
Lenox, MA 01240
1–800–967–3577

Sivananda Yoga Vedanta Center
243 West 24th Street
New York, NY 10011

Call for *Yoga Journal*'s Yoga Teachers Directory,
1–800–359–YOGA

Index

Rosamond Richardson and James Ward are both experienced yoga teachers. Rosamond Richardson is the author of numerous books, and she has appeared on British television as the presenter of BBC2's *Discovering Hedgerows*. The illustrator, James Ward, is a well-known artist and decorative painter.